I0695461

Beauty Without Cosmetics:

361 Natural Home-made Beauty Techniques

By

Timothy M. Ross

Beauty without cosmetics

The publisher's permission must be obtained before duplicating or otherwise reproducing this document. As a result, the information contained therein cannot be transferred electronically, saved in a database, or both. The publisher or creator must give their permission before the document can be copied, scanned, fixed, or stored in any way.

Copyright © by Timothy M. Ross 2023. All rights reserved.

TABLE OF CONTENTS

INTRODUCTION

A beautiful face and skin are attractive indicators of beauty and youth. Shining skin is the craving of all. Time constraint makes beauty care at home difficult. For regeneration and renewal, regrowth and revival, your skin needs time and attention. The quality and tone of your skin would be impossible to improve without basic care. Often we completely ignore the fact that glowing is an indication of our skin being healthy. And healthy skin is the only sure way to have glowing skin. You may buy beauty products, but they work only outside the body. They contain chemicals that are not body-friendly. You don't need harsh chemicals, or endless time to get shiny, healthy hair, smoother skin, and an attractive face. You can go natural. Natural remedies are effective and safe. What you need are some gentle, basic procedures to start looking your best.

The natural beauty materials for glowing skin are what you can make by yourself using herbs, spices, fruits, etc. They work wonders, have lasting results and are inexpensive, what more can anyone ask for. Healthy eating is also crucial. Our face and our hands are important areas on our body that reflect our overall health and well-being. Using simple homemade beauty packs will repair damages from within and give you the desired complexion. You need to realize that protecting your skin from further damage is important too. Otherwise, all your attempts will be of no use as your skin sustains more damage and you will wonder why none of the treatments is showing any results.

Remember, the best beauty secrets are not quick solutions. There are other ingredients of a youthful and beautiful appearance like good sleep, stress-free life, proper nutrition, physical exercise, drinking plenty of water, etc. If you follow these tips consistently the natural herbs can also help you to get rid of wrinkles and aging signs. The beauty materials and methods listed in this book are cheap and natural without negative after-effects.

CHAPTER 1

WHAT PEOPLE WHO USE NATURAL BEAUTY METHODS MUST KNOW AND DO

Cleaning your face and neck with fresh water is a must before using any facial mask.

Remove all cosmetics, creams, and lotions, and use a non abrasive, good-quality beauty soap. Dry your skin with a clean towel after washing your face.

It is preferable to take a hot bath to clean and open up your pores.

Before applying any facial mask, first, take a Patch Test on a little area of your skin and wait for 10 to 15 minutes if it creates an itching or allergic effect then immediately remove it from your skin and avoid the mask.

When you have applied the face mask, lie down, placing a towel under your head and neck. Put 2 cucumber slices on your eyes or use 2 cotton pads soaked in rose water or lavender water.

Do not leave a facial mask on longer than instructed. After the recommended time immediately remove it from your face.

Use a homemade face mask right away after preparing it. However, if you have extra, you can keep most of these facial masks in the refrigerator for up to a week. But always use a freshly made facial mask for the greatest results.

THE BEST FOODS FOR YOUR SKINCARE.

Even beauty experts attach great importance to the following foods:

1. Water(not cold) 3 liters per day. It will make your skin moist and shiny.

2. Green vegetables such as amaranth, broccoli and cabbage contain a lot of vitamins and minerals.

3. Watermelon and cantaloupe provide enough water and nutrition.

4. Lean meat, chicken and fish. They can provide plenty of protein and iron.

5. Coarse food grains and beans. They supply special nutrients needed by the skin.

CHECKLIST OF SKIN BEAUTY CARE

1. Exercise at least three times weekly, even if for 30 mins. It improves skin glow.

2. Don't smoke.

3. Use a natural cleanser and moisturizer.

4. Always remove any makeup, don't leave them overnight.

5. Use rose water as a mild toner, it will leave your skin feeling soft and smooth.

6. Use fresh ripe pawpaw to get glowing skin instantly! Take a small piece of freshly cut ripe pawpaw and gently rub it on your face. Rinse after roughly 15 minutes of leaving it on. You'll see results right away!

7. Each night, wash your face gently with a gentle cleanser before refreshing it with rose water.

8. Each night, wash your face with a gentle cleanser before misting your face with rose water.

9. Using almond oil at night could enable you to wake up with skin that is glowing.

10. If you have sensitive skin, once a week, after opening your pores with warm water and steam, try blending little amounts of castor and body oils into your troublesome acne patches. Even though it might seem counterproductive, this truly helps.

11. Tea tree oil with a 15% concentration works wonders for Acne-prone and blemished skin. Overnight, apply immediately to the acne-affected areas. Though it could dry up your mouth a little, this is completely safe. In the morning, after washing your face, apply a mild moisturizer and your skin will glow.

CHAPTER 2

HERBAL SKIN CARE TIPS FOR SMOOTH, SHINING SKIN

Glowing skin is a major cornerback for women in general. They try different cosmetics to get beautiful and glowing skin. They are unaware that bright skin is a sign of healthy skin. However, your body should deliver nutrients to your skin. Externally applied lotions and creams cannot nourish the skin from the inside. The effects of these medicines are only transient. Chemically created cosmetics, however, have some negative side effects when worn repeatedly. A few natural herbs that work better wonders for your skin. We all secretly desire long, lustrous hair and spotless complexion. An exhaustive list of beauty tips for getting fair skin at home is provided here. It's more than just face packs. Specific foods and other skin care basics that are often ignored or overlooked are equally provided.

Do you want a natural cure that can make your skin seem healthy and radiant? These natural remedies are effective and safe. If you follow these tips consistently you can get healthy shining skin and also get rid of wrinkles and aging signs.

CHAPTER 3

92 NATURAL WAYS TO GET A CLEAR, FAIR COMPLEXION.

1. Eat a Diet that gives Clear Skin: It is the food you eat that ultimately reflects on your face. Your diet provides nutrients for your body for the repair of damaged tissues, mending collagen, building new cells and bones, producing enzymes and proteins, etc. Help your body by eating a diet that includes fruits and vegetables, fiber, lean protein, and complex carbohydrates which are less in saturated fat. Go for berries, the

best food for clear skin, since they contain antioxidants that work to reduce skin aging. Avoid alcohol, smoking and drug abuse, these can cause premature skin aging

2. Drink enough water to maintain your skin well-hydrated from the inside out. Since one of the skin's main jobs is to detoxify the body, doing so is a natural method to get clear skin. Your skin won't glow if you have a lot of trash in your body. Flush out the toxins and waste, drink a lot of water to prevent acne and have clear skin. Be aware that you cannot replace water with drinking beverages containing water, they do not give the same results. Beverages

containing water like coffee, soda, tea and other caffeinated beverages do not help in hydrating the skin rather they remove water from the skin.

3. Workout and wash your face: The main causes of your skin problems are toxins and excessive oil secretion by skin glands. Regular exercise promotes blood circulation throughout the body, including the face, and helps you maintain a healthy weight. When you exercise, your body's pores, particularly those on your face, open up. To remove perspiration and pollutants after working out, take a shower and wash your face. This will help in getting clear skin. During teenage, acne is

developed mainly because of over activity of hormones. Exercising regularly helps to regulate the surge of hormones.

4. As your skin needs to breathe, take off your makeup before bed. When you go to bed wearing makeup, your pores remain clogged all night long, which prevents you from having clear skin.

5. Get enough Sleep: You need adequate sleep to get clear skin, repair damaged tissues and reduce the risk of getting dirt and oil onto your face, it all happens while you sleep. Dirt and oil are the main causes of acne outbreaks. Change your pillow cover at least once a week. The oil, grime,

saliva and dirt stick onto your pillow when you sleep and these in turn get onto your face every time you sleep, which can cause acne breakout. So wash pillow-covers or change them regularly. If you have long hair tie it to the back while you sleep to prevent your hair from touching your face. Once more, this helps prevent acne outbreaks.

6. Maintain good hygiene by washing your face every day, especially in the morning and at night. This aids in clearing the skin and limiting bacterial growth. Before touching or washing your face, wash your hands to avoid transferring any bacteria or dirt from your hands to your face.

Wash your face with a mild cleanser. Never scrub vigorously or rub your face with a scratchy washcloth.

7. To get clear skin, use organic or herbal products instead of chemical products.

8. Picking at your pimples could result in scars; abstain from doing so.

9. HomeMade Exfoliator: Mix two tablespoons of sugar with two tablespoons of water. Stir it thoroughly to make a thin paste and then add one more tablespoon of sugar, and stir again. Wash your hands clean and rub your hands mildly over your face to make it wet.

Scoop up the sugar and water and apply it on one of your cheeks and mildly rub the sugar in circular motions over your other cheek for one minute and then rinse off with clean water. Repeat this process over your other cheek and then to your forehead and the rest of your face.

10. Apply banana with milk on your face and neck, and use it as a beauty tip to get fair, smooth and shining skin.

11. Apply honey for 15 minutes, or use with curd, liquorice, or lemon to get a soft, fair and glowing complexion. Do this daily to replace moisture in your skin.

12. Apply bread crumbs with malai(milk cream) to get fair and smooth skin with glows from within.

13. Soak sunflower seeds (Chirongi) in raw milk overnight and grind them. Use a pinch of each turmeric and saffron when applying. This home beauty tip makes even a dark skin person fairer, and glowing naturally when used for a long time.

14. For naturally fairer, softer, and more radiant skin, combine lentils, curd or milk, lemon juice, and rice. Alternate days for this.

15. Apply egg white and honey for 20 minutes to tighten your skin, make it soft and keep it looking young.

16. To get fairer, boil cabbage or cumin seeds in water. Wash your face with the resulting solution to achieve a radiant shine.

17. To give your face a healthy shine, apply a mixture of mango peels and one spoonful of milk on your face and neck.

18. Combine 1 spoon of sugar with 1 lemon juice. scrub until all the sugar has melted on your body and face. It's a very useful beauty tip for getting soft and fair skin.

19. Apply the mixture of corn flour and egg white to get a glowing and fair complexion.

20. Massage your face with 3 spoons of baby oil, and 2 spoons of sugar daily. This beauty tip gives you a baby soft skin.

21. To acquire naturally smooth, fair, and radiant skin, use malai/milk cream mixed with lemon juice every day.

22. Use 1 spoon of milk, 1 spoon of honey and 1 mashed papaya to get glowing and fair skin naturally.

23. Mix 1/4 part of an orange and 1 spoon of curd to get soft and glowing skin naturally. Quite effective as curd has lactic acid to make you fair, and orange contains vitamin C to nourish your skin.

24. Apply half a spoonful of cinnamon and 2 spoons of honey for fair and smooth skin.

25. Apply raw milk/milk cream to get smooth and fair skin. Mix a pinch of saffron to enhance its effect. Use this beauty tip to clean your face with cotton balls.

26. Rub lemon on your face to get glowing and fair skin. Lemon juice

can also have a tiny bit of turmeric added to it. Lemon has ascorbic acid which tones the skin.

27. Rub orange peels with curd/milk to get fair, soft and glowing skin naturally.

28. To acquire fair, smooth, and beautiful skin, massage almond oil, coconut oil, jojoba oil, mineral oil, or olive oil over your face. Add a pinch of saffron to the oil.

29. Apply aloe vera juice to get naturally soft, glowing skin.

30. To acquire soft, glowing skin naturally, use a mixture of 2 spoons

of rose water, 1/2 spoon of glycerin, sunflower oil, and sugar.

31. Apply a mixture of banana, honey, potato and bergamot oil for 20 minutes to remove pigmentations or marks from your face. Potato is a natural fairness agent.

32. To acquire clean, radiant skin, steam your face while adding mint leaves, lavender, peppermint, or chamomile to two glasses of water. Do this once in 15 days. If you have acne on your face this remedy works.

33. Cleanse your face every day with gram flour or fuller's earth (multani mitti), neem (margosa), and licorice.

For dry skin, combine all the ingredients with milk cream; for oily skin, combine with cucumber. It's an ideal daily beauty procedure for face cleaning.

34. Apply corn flour or oatmeal with cucumber juice to tighten the pores.

35. Scrub your face with a mixture of one spoonful of curd, two spoons of barley flour, and a little bit of turmeric. It will give you fair, soft and glowing skin.

36. Apply curd and turmeric as a beauty tip for hair and glowing skin.

37. Apply almond powder, milk cream and rose petals together to get a rose-like glow and softness to your complexion.

38. Apply 1 spoon of clay powder with 1 spoon of honey on your face. Wash off with warm water to get smooth and glowing skin naturally.

39. Apply tomato and honey on your face for 20 mins to get fair, soft and oil-free skin.

40. Mix 250gms of milk powder, half a cup of almond oil and any essential oil in water. Soak yourself in this water to look soft and glowing.

41. Use milk, peeled almonds, a pinch of barley flour, a pinch of turmeric and 1 spoon of honey to get glowing and wrinkle-free skin.

42. Apply lemon and cucumber daily to get oil-free, fair and glowing complexion.

43. Apply cucumber and curd for 20 minutes for glowing and oil-free skin.

44. Mix 1 tsp buttermilk with 1 tsp radish juice to reduce wrinkles and skin roughness.

45. Apply sandalwood with milk to get glowing, smooth and fair skin at home.

46. Apply raw milk with lemon juice to tighten the open pores.

47. Mix 2 spoons of soy flour, 1 and a half spoon curd and a spoon of honey to rejuvenate wrinkled and dull skin. Use this effective beauty tip to tighten sagged skin.

48. Rub watermelon on the skin to get soft, glowing and fair skin.

49. Mix 2 spoons of barley flour, 1 spoon of honey and a half cup of ripe pawpaw and use to get a soft, fair, and glowing complexion.

50. Mix cabbage juice, half a spoon of barley flour and 1 spoon of honey, and apply on your face to get fair, smooth and radiant skin.

51. Rub on pears mixed with half a spoon of lemon juice and tomato juice to get beautiful and fair skin.

52. Use the powder of 2 almonds, 1 spoon of carrot juice and 1 spoon of orange juice on the skin for 15 mins to remove scars and pigmentations.

53. Apply apple juice with lemon juice(half part apple juice) to get a glow in your skin.

54. Use amla oil (Indian gooseberry oil) mixed with glycerin for a beautiful soft and glowing complexion.

55. Apply black gram (urad daal) with the powder of 4 almonds as a natural toner to make your complexion fair and soft.

56. Apply pineapple juice to clean your face and combat aging.

57. Apply carrot juice with 1 spoon of honey to brighten your complexion. Wash off with water mixed with baking soda. You can add pawpaw to the mixture.

58. To revive the lifeless and pale skin, dab on a half-spoon of almond powder, two spoons of barley flour, and rose water.

59. Apply curd and walnut powder as a home remedy to get a glow in your face naturally at home.

60. Apply 2 spoons of honey with 2 spoons of lemon juice and powdered almonds for 30 minutes to get fair, glowing and soft skin.

61. Use the mixture of egg yolk, 2 spoons of almond oil and 1 ripe banana to get soft, fair and glowing skin.

62. Apply fuller earth and sandalwood for beautiful, fair, smooth and glowing skin.

63. Use gram flour, curd/milk and lemon juice to get smooth, fair and glowing skin.

64. Mix malai with 1 spoonful of walnut powder, honey and lemon juice to scrub your face for 20 mins. It gives soft, fair and glowing skin.

65. Turmeric mixed with orange juice works as a good scrub. Use this for 20 minutes to give you fair and glowing skin.

66. Rub pawpaw or avocado for 15 minutes to get a radiant and glowing complexion.

67. Mix banana, lemon juice, honey and margarine together to make a mask. Leave overnight on the face, hands and feet. Then wash off to get fair and glowing skin.

68. Cucumber with coconut water is an excellent skin treatment for getting fair, soft and glowing skin. It will remove scars even chicken pot scars from the face.

69. Boil orange peels in the water to use as a toner.

70. Diet- Drink a lot of water to get a fair, smooth and glowing complexion from within. Drink fruit juice to clear your blood. Eat apples, guava, pears, vegetables, fish, eggs, nuts, oatmeal, melons, carrots, etc. Drink milk with a pinch of saffron and drink amla juice daily. Take a blood purifier daily.

71. Morning FACE Beauty Treatment: Using ice cubes on the face every morning freshens and rejuvenates the skin but it is a little harsh. Rather, simply wipe your face in the morning with cold raw milk. Additionally, you can combine milk and cucumber juice, then use a cotton ball to apply the mixture to your face.

Rinse your face with cold water afterward. This freshens your face, cleans your skin and leaves your face fresh.

72. Make your hands beautiful using coffee: The coffee you drink can be used for skin care also, ground coffee is a natural exfoliator. Exfoliation removes dead and dry skin cells from the skin's surface and boosts the natural skin renewal process, making your skin look healthy and smooth, try this good beauty recipe, mix grounded coffee with olive oil(or any other oil of your choice, avoid using petroleum based oils, use natural oils and massage your hands in a circular motion, with this homemade hand

scrub for a few minutes, rinse your hands with lukewarm water. You'll notice how delicate and gentle your hands feel. Your hands will appear appealing if you do this twice a week.

73. Effective natural BODY scrub recipe: For a homemade body scrub: Mix 2 tablespoons of used coffee grounds, 1 tablespoon of sugar and 4 tablespoons of olive oil. Massage your body with this scrub while in the shower, applying it in circular motions, especially concentrating on the areas with fatty deposits, on your legs and on dry areas of your body. You will notice its amazing effect on your skin.

74. Good Beauty Habits. Wash your face at night. During the day, makeup dirt and oil build up on your face. Include skin cleansing in your bedtime routine. Use makeup remover to avoid spreading bacteria to your pillow and preventing it from clogging your pores and triggering breakouts as you sleep, If your skin feels tight and dry after washing, you're using too powerful of a cleanser where it can penetrate into your skin and not totally strip it of all oils. The skin around the eyes can be too fragile for most cleansers, so avoid the eye area. To get rid of the cleanser, sprinkle some water on your face. Your skin may get even more irritated if you clean it up with a rag

or washcloth. Instead, bend your face over the sink, cup your hands together and bring up small amounts of water to splash over your face. It should only take ten splashes, then pat dry. Drying your skin with a towel shouldn't be done in a hard manner; instead, use little, delicate pats or let it air dry.

75. Exfoliate once a week: If your skin tends to be dry and flaky, a weekly exfoliation can clear out dead skin cells. An effective exfoliant is a straightforward sugar and honey scrub. With warm water, rinse it off. A face-specific dry brush is another option for exfoliation. Make tiny,

circular movements as you brush your face.

76. Protect your skin from the sun: Avoid leathery, tough skin by avoiding the hot blare of the sun. Avoid sun damage and keep your skin supple for many years.

77. Eat Healthy and Exercise Regularly: Don't stop drinking water: You need 3 liters of water a day. The water will clear your skin and make it shine as it helps your body to flush out toxins quickly. Carry a water bottle with you all day to ensure you have water.

78. Drink Green Tea or other juices to hydrate when you're tired of water. Eat a healthy diet. Nutritional fruits and vegetables, lean proteins, and healthy fats all contribute to glowing skin. Add these gods to your diet to see quick results.

79. Omega 3 fatty acids: Found in fish, pear and walnuts are beneficial to the skin.

80. Vitamin C helps your pimples heal faster, so eat some citrus fruits and spinach.

81. Fiber-rich foods, Fresh vegetables, nuts and unprocessed fruit help keep a fine balance and be

regular, not sluggish, in the gastrointestinal area. You may look and feel tired and sickly (headache and abdominal complaints) if you do not have regularity of elimination/ movements once or more every day.

82. Avoid sugar and eat less salt: Eating too much salt can make your face look bloated.

83. Take vitamins, If you're worried you aren't getting enough of the necessary vitamins and minerals, try taking a multivitamin they are beneficial to the skin.

84. Exercise regularly: It makes your skin glow as it stimulates blood flow.

It's also healthy for the body and makes you stronger. Reap short and long-term benefits.

85. Excessive production of Melanin Pigment gives the skin a dark complexion and the hotter your environment the more it is produced. Applying a mixture of sandalwood and Rose water cools your skin as well as brings a fair glow to you.

86. Applying a paste of finely ground almonds and rose water regularly on the face and neck gives a Natural Fairness.

87. Soak four almonds overnight. In the morning remove the skins and

grind them fine. Add one teaspoon of milk and four drops of lime juice, and mix all. Regular massage with this paste gives natural fair skin.

88. Vegetables are the best natural way to achieve fairness. Simply Cut a tomato into two halves and rub it on your face. You can see the change within a few days. Alternatively, you might give potatoes a 10-minute soak in cold water. Rub the slices on your face, hands and neck. Do it regularly to bring a positive result within a short period.

89. You can make a paste of cucumber with coconut water. Apply

this paste regularly to get a fair and glowing complexion.

90. Apply a mixture of equal amounts of lemon and cucumber juice on the face and whole body. 15 minutes after applying, rinse it off. This will also help you to increase fair color.

91. Apply the turmeric powder and sandalwood paste daily to get a fair color.

92. Rose Oil is a cooling agent against the production of Melanin pigment and a natural way to give you fair and glowing skin. It contains plenty of vitamins C and E, which are necessary for having younger-looking

skin. Rose oil removes dead cells from the skin and provides relief from burns, slowing the aging process. Rose oil is used for cleansing, toning, moisturizing and nourishing the skin.

CHAPTER 4

9 UNBELIEVABLE BEAUTY TIPS

1. To Make Your Teeth Whiter.

You need dental floss and baking soda. Do this once a month, it's very hard on the teeth, but an effective natural teeth whitener. Brush and rinse as usual. Apply baking soda on your teeth's flat surfaces. Use the dental floss to create a mini sander between your teeth, be sure to get into the gum a bit. Apply baking soda on your teeth's flat surfaces. Do the same for upper teeth. Brush your teeth and rinse again.

2. Face Mask.

If you're all dried out from the cold, dry heat, try this incredible natural mask to help the dryness caused by other artificial products.

• Half cup powdered oats (powder in a blender)

• 2 tbsp honey

• 1 squished gel-cap of vitamin E

• 1 teaspoon sunflower oil or any type of liquid oil

• If your skin is affected, DO NOT use half a teaspoon of vanilla extract.

• To create a paste, add water. Warm compresses warm the skin and open the pores. Apply the mixture to your skin and leave it there for at least 10 minutes. On typically dry regions, rinse and apply a small amount of liquid vegetable oil.

3. Pimple Relief.
To remove pimples quickly, try this natural approach.
Hot compress, 10 minutes. Cool compress for 10 minutes.
Do another hot compress. Gently expel the pimple if it has come to a head. If you tried and it wouldn't come out, apply another hot compress

and another cold compress to reduce the swelling.

Repeat the hot/cold procedure the next night if the pimple is extremely large. Make a paste out of a tiny bit of baking soda and some water in the evening if the pimple is close to the surface. Apply a small amount on the pimple and cover it with a bandage to keep the baking soda in place. The following morning ought to be better. Baking soda removes part of the oil from the pimple while also eradicating bacteria. Do the hot /cold compresses again the next night and it should pop out, if not, do the baking soda again.

4. Blackheads Can Disappear.

Natural methods are the simplest and most affordable for getting rid of blackheads. Try this all-natural, non-toxic technique to treat your blackhead issues. It's effective! To open the pores and soften the blackhead, apply warm compresses. They won't leave scars, so gently pop them out. Make more compresses if they don't come out easily. Wash well with organic soap. Use witch hazel or lemon juice to clean. To lessen redness, apply a cool compress.

5. Proper moisturizer
Try this all-natural technique for a long-lasting moisturizer that penetrates deeply and helps feed your cells.

To soften skin tissue and widen pores, apply warm compresses. Any natural vegetable oil, such as extra-virgin olive oil, sunflower oil, or coconut oil, should be generously applied. Lay the heated compress on your moisturized skin for around 10 minutes. Rinse after washing with a natural soap. You will undoubtedly notice and experience the effect that going natural has on your skin.

6. Cuticle (Nail) health
You Need; 2 Tablespoon cooking oil Natural soap and Toothpick Remove nail polish. For a thorough cleaning and cuticle softening, wash your hands in warm water with natural soap. drier hands. On each fingernail,

gently massage some cooking oil. Make sure you apply oil to your fingernails' whole surface. You can clean between your nails with a toothpick. Again, use a natural soap and warm water to wash your hands. Everywhere around each fingernail, massage the cuticle with a toothpick.

7. Exfoliant and Natural Dermabrasion

Chemical and mechanical dermabrasion are the two available techniques. Chemical dermabrasion harms the outermost layers of skin, resulting in skin peeling. Simply said, mechanical dermabrasion removes the outermost layers of skin using a coarse lubricant. You should consider choosing only mechanical methods of dermabrasion that are gentle on the skin but will bring out a natural healthy glow. What you need, Powdered flowers, oats, bananas, essential oils, or herbs or use what you like.

Basic Dermabrasion-

1 tablespoon baking soda

Warm water to moisten skin

Wet skin. Gently exfoliate your skin with baking soda using your hands or a washcloth. Baking soda eliminates oils and dead skin cells while also killing bacteria. Rinse.

8. Girl area' bump reducer

The hairs in this area are being removed beneath the skin's surface, resulting in bumps. Conventional body care products aggravate skin because they include chemicals that are overly potent and can result in contact dermatitis symptoms, such as an enlargement of the cells around recently shaved hair. Choose to use a new razor, a natural soap without ingredients you can't pronounce, and follow with a hazel wipe to kill bacteria and reduce swelling of the tissue caused by irritation from shaving.

9. Relaxing bath blend
I love long, hot, relaxing baths. Here are a few items you can put in your

tub to make a bath much more pleasant than just soaking in plain water.

1 cup powdered oats

2 cups Dead Sea salt

1 cup Epsom salt

3 tablespoons vanilla extract

2 tablespoons of vegetable oil, e.g. extra-virgin olive oil, sunflower, or coconut oil. Add to your hot bath water. Enter in with a book and enjoy it.

CHAPTER 5

17 ASSORTED NATURAL BEAUTY IDEAS

1. Many wrinkles, pimples, and even creases in the cleavage area can be avoided by sleeping on your back.
2. Dressing in tight clothing gives you a heavier appearance. Even a skinny female might develop a bulge under too-tight clothing.
3. Getting upset will make you look older and more wrinkled later on.
4. Less makeup helps you appear younger.
5. While more isn't necessarily better when it comes to vitamins and minerals, they are essential for good

health and beauty. Selenium or Vitamin A excess might lead to hair loss.

6. If you are unhappy with a hair conditioner, it will still make a good "shaving cream" for your legs in the shower.

7. Avoid stretching the skin during shaving to prevent ingrown hairs from being triggered by shaving the hair just slightly under the skin.

8. Drink a lot of water and get enough sleep daily as part of a beauty regime.

9. To maintain a youthful, bouncy bosom, tighten bra straps when they sag or get a new bra when they can no longer be made any tighter.

10. Instead of repeatedly shaving, which causes the hairs to grow

thicker and darker each time, try waxing. After a few sessions, irreversible hair loss will ensue from waxing, which causes softer hairs each time.

11. Sleeping on two or three pillows at a time or putting a wedge pillow under your regular pillow will help get rid of dark circles under your eyes.

12. Exercise while dieting is a must or your skin will be too large and saggy for your smaller body. It is tougher to tighten skin after your body shrinks.

13. After washing your face, rinse in cold water(fair-skinned people should use cool instead of cold) to close the

pores and tighten the skin after your body shrinks.

14. You can look considerably slimmer if you have good posture.

15. If you wear low heels as opposed to flats, your posture will be better.

16. Excessive use of very high heels will result in a masculine, chiseled calf as opposed to a feminine, rounded calf.

17. Occasionally wash hair brushes with dish soap and borax. In a dishpan of very warm water, add half a cup of borax and a few drops of liquid dish soap. The brushes should be stirred, rinsed, and allowed to air dry. Utilize a worn-out toothbrush to scrub any tough locations.

CHAPTER 6

8 NATURAL BEAUTY METHODS FOR DARK SKIN

1. Orange Mask for Black skin:
Make a paste by grinding some orange peels. Mix it with homemade yogurt. Now apply this paste to your face and hands. Leave it for 20 to 30 minutes and then wash with lukewarm water. Apply regularly.
2. Turmeric Mask for Black Skin:
Apply a mixture of yogurt, lime juice, and turmeric powder on the area that is colored. Keep this paste for at least 10 lines and wash it with fresh water. To get faster results, do it every day.
3. Potato for Black Skin:

Potato paste is a wonderful bleaching agent. Apply a paste on your skin and keep it for at least half an hour and then wash it with water.

4. Almonds

This also makes the skin healthy and shining. Take 2 or 3 almonds, soak them in water overnight, and then make a paste of it. Apply the paste on your face and keep it until it dries and then wash it with cold water.

5. Mix cucumber juice and honey all together:

Apply on the face and keep it until the paste dries, then wash it off. Do it at least once a week to get a better result.

6. Do not attempt to change your skin color:

However, you can make your skin problem-free and shining.

7. Balanced diet:

In addition to using various products, you also have to maintain a good balanced diet. Include lots of fresh fruits and vegetables loaded with vitamins in your meal.

8. Drinking lots of fluids like fresh water and various fruit juices is also necessary to have glowing skin.

CHAPTER 7

10 SUPER SIMPLE NATURAL BEAUTY TIPS

1. Banana and Egg Hair Treatment
Give your hair a little more shine. Combine one egg with mashed banana. It should be applied to your hair as a thick paste and left on for 10 to 30 minutes. Wash it off.
2. Moisturizing Nail Treatment
Admire your lovely hands after soaking your nails in olive oil for five minutes.
3. Simple Honey Face Mask
Raw honey is naturally antibacterial and a quick way to get soft, beautiful skin. Use a spoonful of unprocessed

raw honey once each week, and gently warm it between your hands. Cover your face with it. Use warm water to gently rinse it off after leaving it on for 5 to 10 minutes, then pat dry.

4. Apple Cider Vinegar Clarifying Shampoo

If you use commercial shampoos you may need to eliminate any buildup in your hair, mix half a cup of organic apple cider vinegar (like this) with 1 cup of water. Follow with your usual conditioner.

5. Elbow and Knee Exfoliate and Skin Brightener.

Cut an orange into half and rub it on your elbows and knees. It has a pleasant scent and helps to smooth down those rough places. Rinse off the sticky mess.

6. Gentle Body Scrub

To create a quick and efficient body scrub, use sea salt and olive oil in a 2 to 1 ratio. Dead skin cells are removed as a result, leaving behind smoother, more radiant skin. And compared to pricey body scrubs from the shop, this natural beauty tip is significantly more affordable.

7. Easy Deep Conditioning Hair Treatment

If you want very soft, hydrated hair, use melted coconut oil as a deep conditioner for hair and scalp treatment. After massaging coconut oil into your scalp, rub your fingers through your hair. Leave it on for a couple of hours and then wash it out using shampoo, coconut oil will saturate your hair with awesome goodness, It may be extremely difficult to remove with simply baking soda and organic shampoos. Before doing this, you might want to see if you can remove it with a small amount of coconut oil on a small part of your hair. Otherwise, you might have greasy(but soft!) hair for a few washings.

8. Simple Toxic-Free Shaving Cream
As a natural alternative to shaving cream, apply coconut oil to your legs.

9. All Natural Black Head Removal
A lemon wedge should have 4 or 5 drops of raw honey on it. Next, rub the lemon for a minute on your face,

paying special attention to any problem areas. After five minutes, remove the liquid and rinse with cold water. It is advisable to do this before night rather than before going out because citrus might make your skin photosensitive.

10. Dry Brushing for Better Skin
Your body may easily cleanse using the dry-brushing technique. Through a light massage, it stimulates several organs. Additionally, it supports the lymphatic system, gets rid of dead skin cells and immune system buildup, boosts hormone production, can get rid of cellulite, and can help tighten skin by improving circulation. What's more, it's quick and affordable.

Keep in mind that the best beauty tricks are not fast solutions. They need sufficient sleep, effective stress management, a healthy diet, and regular exercise. Although all of the aforementioned "gems" can help your beauty regimen to some extent, keep in mind that true beauty is the product of everyday body care. And by being you.

CHAPTER 8

15 WAYS TO USE FRUITS TO ENHANCE YOUR NATURAL BEAUTY

1. Grapes:

Grapes are highly beneficial for your skin. It can be used to physically cleanse your skin or you can juice them and apply the juice to your skin. This will give you smooth, radiant skin. Grapes Mask: To make your face bright and shiny, take a few grapes and rub them on your face, or make it into a pack by mashing the grapes.

2. Cucumber Juice, Glycerine, and Rose Water:

An effective combination is rose water, glycerin, and cucumber juice. Use it before going out in the sun and when you come back. Apply it to your skin and then rinse it off after 15 minutes. This mixture protects your skin from sun damage.

3. Sandalwood, Turmeric and Milk: Sandalwood powder, a little turmeric powder, and milk are combined to form a fine paste. Utilize milk to blend this substance. You should apply this paste to your skin and leave it on for five minutes. Your skin would seem healthy and radiant as a result.

4. Honey and Cream:

An excellent technique to maintain the skin soft and radiant, especially during the dry season, is to combine honey and cream. Mix some honey with cream and apply to your face. This would make your skin moist, soft, and bright.

5. Fresh Milk, Salt and Lime Juice: Get some fresh milk, add a pinch of salt and a little juice, and apply this mixture to your face. This would open up the pores in your skin and clean out all the debris.

6. Tomato Juice:
Lemon juice and tomato juice together maintain a delicate and radiant complexion. For glowing and healthy skin apply a mixture of tomato juice and lemon juice.

7. Sesame Oil, Wheat Flour, and Turmeric Powder:
For removing facial hair apply a mixture of turmeric powder, sesame oil, and wheat flour. Combine the turmeric powder, wheat flour, and sesame oil to create a paste. To get rid of unwanted hair, apply this to your skin.

8. Cabbage Juice and Honey:
Wrinkles can be avoided by applying some honey and cabbage juice to the face. For preventing wrinkles apply a mixture of cabbage juice and honey.

9. Carrot Juice:
An excellent approach to achieve a natural glow is to directly apply carrot juice to the face.

10. Honey and Cinnamon Powder:

3 parts honey and 1 part cinnamon powder should be combined to form a paste. Apply it on your skin. Let it remain overnight. This is a great treatment for pimples. It also helps remove the scars left by pimples.

11. Groundnut Oil and Lime Juice: To avoid acne and blackheads, combine a little groundnut oil with fresh lime juice and apply it to the face.

12. Aloe Vera Juice: Aloe Vera juice applied to the troublesome regions hydrates the skin while minimizing pigmentation spots.

13. Ghee and Glycerin: A fantastic homemade moisturizer is prepared from ghee and glycerin.

14. Multani Mitti, Rose Petals, Neem, Tulsi, and Rose Water:

The skin is left bright and healthy after being applied with a paste made of multani mitti, rose petals, neem leaf powder, and tulsi leaf powder.

15. Apricots and Yogurt:

To make a paste, combine yogurt and apricots. This improves the skin and gives it a radiant appearance. If your skin is dry, add honey to the mixture. Apply the paste to get fresh-looking skin.

CHAPTER 9

SKINCARE BASICS THAT ENSURE YOUNG-LOOKING SKIN

Whatever beauty regime you adopt, it is important to protect your skin from damage. Otherwise, your best attempts will be ineffective because your skin damage persists and you wonder why none of the beauty treatments are working. For regeneration and renewal, your skin needs time and attention. Without basic care, it would be challenging to improve the health and tone of your skin. These commonly ignored simple daily Skin Care basics will transform your efforts.

A. Drink Lots of Water

Make it a habit to drink a minimum of 3 liters of water daily. For the body to function properly, water is necessary. There is fluid loss from the body due to evaporation, sweating, and urination. The loss must be replenished by drinking plenty of water and homemade juices but not soft drinks. When water intake is less than water loss, dehydration takes place. Generally, fluid loss takes place in warmer climates, among those who do grueling exercises, at high altitudes, and in older people whose sense of thirst has reduced.

You gain energy from water and experience weariness relief. Your face appears incredibly lifeless when you are fatigued and dehydrated. The skin mirrors your health, so you should treat water like a nutrient and drink it. Water doesn't make wrinkles go away, but it does keep your skin hydrated. Water helps digestion and keeps your skin clear and acne-free.

B. Sleep Well

Lack of sleep is evident on your face. You appear irritated and worn out. Avoid skipping out on beauty sleep and avoid staying up late at night to solve the problem. Dark circles are a result of blood vessels expanding due to sleep deprivation. While you sleep, the skin heals, regenerates, and rebalances. The face instantly lifts as the older, healthier skin cells replace the dead ones. The body goes through all of these hormonal and metabolic changes when you sleep. So sleep deprivation interferes with bodily functions. You must get seven to eight hours of sleep each night if you want healthy skin. To avoid cell disintegration, do not oversleep; instead, keep a healthy equilibrium.

C. Exercise

You must exercise for at least 30 minutes every day. Take appropriate measures before exercising if you have skin conditions like acne, psoriasis, or rosacea, but don't allow these to stop you from living an active life. Dermatologists say that exercise helps to increase blood circulation which boosts skin health. Exercise helps remove cellular debris, and free radicals from the body and cleanses it from within. Stress can occasionally increase sebum production from the sebaceous glands, which can lead to skin conditions including eczema and acne. Exercise relieves stress, which prevents skin issues. Exercise most crucially shapes your physique and improves your appearance.

D. Exfoliate

Follow a good skin routine. Do not skip exfoliation as without this, you cannot get rid of dead and dry skin that accumulates and makes your complexion appear dull. You don't need to buy a scrub. Homemade scrubs are just as effective. As an alternative to using a packaged product, use oatmeal. There are many natural options available.

E. Remove Makeup before Sleep

It's crucial to let your skin breathe. Every night before bed, take off your makeup. Do not fail to do this every night no matter how tired you may be. With your makeup on, your skin cannot repair itself.

Perhaps a better method for removing makeup than using harsh chemicals is to use oil. Those with oily skin may think that excess oil can cause more harm, but it is not so. While keeping the skin's natural oils intact, oil helps in the dissolution of impurities and sebum. Those with oily skin can also use a natural cleanser. Make sure the cleanser is water-based. But virgin olive oil is the best, it removes all eye and face makeup in one step. You can also use castor oil, it is antibacterial and good for the skin. You can also blend castor oil and almond oil, avocado oil, and jojoba oil to remove wrinkles and give your skin a natural glow.

Castor oil and half a cup of virgin olive oil are blended. Apply and gently massage on your face, use the oil to remove eye makeup gently. Now dip a washcloth in warm water and wring out the excess moisture. Place it on your face and keep it for a minute, then wipe out the excess oil. This simple oil-cleansing routine will remove all impurities.

F. Eat Vitamin Rich Foods

Include foods high in vitamin A and vitamin C in your diet. As a result, your skin will develop radiant health. Vitamin C tablets are also available. For a clear skin tone, you can take one pill after lunch every day.

CHAPTER 10

HOMEMADE BEAUTY TIPS FOR FAIR SKIN

1. Tea Water and Honey Face Pack: You can use tea water for a bath and soak in its fragrance or you can put tea water in a spray bottle and gently spray it on your face to feel rejuvenated. Utilize regular black tea, green tea, or herbal teas such as chamomile, mint, and lavender. The way you drink tea to relieve stress, similarly de-stress your skin with tea water wash. Your skin will be cleansed of pollutants and free radicals thanks to the antioxidants in tea water.

2. Use Honey to Protect your Face from Bacteria and Keep it Hydrated.
What you need: 1 cup of tea water(Cooled down) 2 spoons of rice flour, and half a spoon of honey(rice flour is an excellent scrub and honey moisturizes the skin).
Procedures: Mix the above ingredients and apply on the skin. Leave it on till the mask dries completely for about 20 minutes or more. Before washing off the mask with water, make sure you massage in circular motions; this is important as it removes the dead skin and evens out the skin tone. Wash your face with cold water. You have a fairer, more even skin tone as a result.

3. Oats and Lemon Face Pack:
Oats are natural exfoliators. Oats are suitable for those who have eczema. If you eat oats for your breakfast to become slim, you can also use them on your skin to clear it of excess oil, grime and impurities. Lemon has skin-lightening qualities and is high in vitamin C. Many commercial fairness creams contain lemon extracts but it is better to use lemon juice directly than using extracts. Avoid giving your skin harsh chemicals.

What you need: 1 tablespoon of oats, cooked and mashed (helps reduce inflammation and heals the skin). 1 tablespoon of lemon juice (lemon helps lighten the skin tone). If you have sensitive skin, you can dilute the lemon juice with water.

Method: Mix the above ingredients and apply on the face by massaging into the skin. Let it dry for 20 minutes. Wash and pat dry.

4. Turmeric and Lemon Face Pack: Perhaps the finest treatment for fair skin is turmeric. Indian Brides look more gorgeous after the turmeric treatment as part of their wedding preparation. Turmeric also gives the skin a visible glow. Turmeric is a very exfoliating agent and also prevents the skin from aging. Additionally, turmeric eliminates wrinkles, blemishes, stretch marks, and acne.

Adding lemon juice to turmeric makes it a potent skin fairness agent. What you need: Gram flour, Turmeric, Lemon juice, and Milk. **Procedure:** Mix the ingredients and apply evenly on the face. Gently scrub the paste for five minutes, then wait 20 minutes for it to dry. Clean your face.

5. Turmeric and Tomato Face Pack: An antioxidant called lycopene guards against sun damage to the face. It is also an excellent anti-aging agent. So stay young with a tomato diet.

What you need: Turmeric, Tomato juice.

Procedure: Mix turmeric with tomato juice. Apply it on your face, then give it time to dry. Wash your face with warm water. This is a popular pack among women because it is simple and gives good results. You might also remove the tomato pulp and use it to massage your skin. It should be rinsed out after 15 to 20 minutes. If you do this every day, it will assist your complexion later.

6. Turmeric Face Pack:

This is an all-time favorite. The results have always been so stunning that this has now become a must-do ritual for a bride before the wedding day.

What you need: Gram flour (good exfoliator), Pinch of turmeric (lightens skin tone), Milk(moisturizer).
Method: Mix the ingredients and apply the mask. Gently scrub the paste for five minutes, then wait 20 minutes for it to dry. Once it's dry, clean your face.

7. Yogurt and dried orange peel: Orange is rich in vitamin C and it is a good skin tonic. It keeps other skin issues at bay while aiding in the treatment and prevention of acne. Yogurt is the best thing you can do for your skin. It is good for your health and it makes your skin glow. Plain yogurt fights acne, skin

discoloration, and signs of aging like fine lines and wrinkles. The best thing about yogurt is that it is the most effective moisturizer for all skin. What you need: Dried orange peel, fresh and unflavored yogurt, Dry the orange peels first under the sun before grinding.

8. Yogurt and Lemon:
Yogurt and lemon both hydrate skin and get rid of imperfections that give the face a lifeless appearance. The combination will add shine to your face.
What you need: Fresh and unflavored yogurt, and fresh lemon juice.

Method: Mix 1 teaspoon of lemon juice with 1 tablespoon of fresh and unflavored yogurt and mix well, apply and keep on cleansed skin for 15-20 minutes, then rinse off. Your skin will become fairer as a result, and any acne scars and dark patches on your skin will fade away.

9. Milk, Lemon Juice and Honey: The combination of raw milk, honey and lemon will make you fair naturally, it will also lock moisture in your skin. Your skin will be shielded physically from external elements like pollutants that could harm it.
What you need: Milk, Lemon Juice, Honey.

Method: Use 1 tsp. each of milk/milk powder, honey and lemon juice, and mix to form a paste. It should be applied on cleansed skin and left for 15-20 minutes. You may then rinse it off.

10. Milk and Saffron:

The best ingredient for skin fairness is said to be saffron. It is more expensive than other food items but is worth investing in saffron to get the golden glow.

What you need: Cold, milk(raw)- 2 to 3 teaspoons, a few strands of saffron.

Method: Put 5-6 strands of saffron in the milk. Let it stay for 3-4 hours.

After washing your face and neck, apply this mixture. Leave it on for 15-20 minutes. Wash off with lukewarm water. This is an effective means to achieve fairness. It also makes skin soft and smooth. Raw milk is not heavy, hence, it suits all skin types.

11. Pawpaw and Fuller's Earth: Papaya and fuller's earth or multani mitti make the skin fair and healthy. Both are popularly used in many beauty products but a natural homemade mask protects your skin from chemicals. Oily-skinned people can use this face pack too.

What you need: 1 tbsp. pawpaw pulp, 1 teaspoon fuller's earth.

Method: Mix the two together, apply on cleansed skin, let it dry and rinse off.

12. Potato:

After peeling potatoes, save the skin since it can be used as a scrub. You can also grate or make potato juice and use it for your skin. All debris and dead skin cells are removed, leaving your skin looking young and healthy.

What you need: Potato slices, in pulp or juice form.

Method: Use potato slices or the paste of potato as a mask or you can even apply the juice on dark portions of the skin. This can be applied twice daily on your skin. Use plain water to rinse off after 15 to 20 minutes.

13. Lemon or Orange Rind:
This citrus combination will do wonders to your skin because of its high vitamin C content. It will brighten and protect your skin. You can use it to solve acne and other skin problems as well.
What you need: Lemon or orange rind, Raw milk.
Method: Take lemon rind(grated outer skin), or even orange, dry them under the sun (do not microwave) and then grind them to powder.
Store in a dry air-tight container, mix it with raw milk and use as a pack on the affected areas. Wash off with

warm water only. Immediately use a cooling toner.

14. Healthy Diet:

With daily care treatments taken care of, what you need to monitor next is your eating habits. Without the right nutrients, your skin cannot undo the damage that it sustains every day. The right quantities of all the ingredients need to be consumed for the skin to be healthy and for fairness to be reflected. Consume vitamin C-rich fruits to benefit from the antioxidants they hold. Balance your diet to get the right amount of proteins and unsaturated fats along with fresh, green vegetables to provide the right portions of nutrients for your skin to naturally care for itself.

15. Sun Protection and Care:
Avoid the hot sun, sun rays and UV radiation have damaging effects on your skin.

CHAPTER 11

26 UNCOMMON METHODS TO GET SHINING SKIN

1. Harsh Sun Rays is no Friend to the Skin:
Avoiding overexposure to the sun is the single easiest way to look younger for life. Ninety percent of wrinkles are from sun exposure, it's so much easier to prevent the damage than to cure it later.

2. Clean your Makeup Brushes. According to a British survey, 72% of women never wash their brushes or sponges, despite the fact that they accumulate dirt and bacteria that might result in breakouts. Brushes for

loose powder should be washed every two weeks.

3. Eat Mixed Nuts:

Brazil nuts increase skin elasticity and prevent skin cancer, according to recent studies. Then walnuts, loaded with omega 3 fatty acids- to lower inflammation and stop breakouts. High-grade oils and fatty acids found in macadamias help to rejuvenate and restore skin.

4. Sanitize your Mobile Phones:

According to a Stanford University Study, the iPhone gets more germ-infested than a public toilet. In fact, distributing viruses on mobile devices may be nearly as harmful as sneezing in someone's face due to the glass touch screens' propensity for doing so. Every time you make a call, all those germs land directly on your cheek and jawline, resulting in spots and irritation. Wipe your phone (and face) down many times per day with an antibacterial wipe, such as Clorox Disinfecting Wipes, to keep them free of bacteria.

5. Apply your Beauty Materials in the Proper Order:

It's possible that the order in which you use your products could be even more crucial than the products themselves. As soon as you wash and pat your skin dry, choose products with the most active components. These are the most powerful, so you want them to come into direct contact with your skin, anything that's water soluble should go first, followed by the product that's thicker and creamier. Reverse the process, and the heavier cream will prevent the lighter cream's components from reaching the skin and having any effect.

6. Avoid Dairy in the Diet:

Dairy Products. Even those that are organic, contain cow hormones that stimulate your oil glands and your pores, leading to acne. Be careful of Dairy foods, Ike salad dressing, protein bars and shakes. Stick to skimmed milk. Fat is your greatest choice because the hormones are concentrated there.

7. Get Adequate Sleep:

It is called beauty sleep. Sleep deprivation lowers circulation, which is why you look dull and washed out if you don't get enough. The optimum moment to renew your skin is also now. Your body's cellular renewal teamwork in the night, so equip your skin with as many nutrients and hydrating ingredients it needs to do a fine job.

8. Exfoliate for Smaller-looking Pores:

One of the most frequent concerns about beauty is enlarged pores, which is astonishing considering how small something can seem. When pores are clogged with debris, oil, dead skin cells, and the skin protein keratin, they seem larger. Those plugs appear to shrink when removed. To clear out the dirt, start exfoliating regularly.

Avoid the sun to prevent pores from getting even larger as you age. Collagen is broken down by sun exposure, and this has an impact on pore size as well.

9. Don't Neglect your Neck and Chest:

Many stop their skincare routine at the chin. Neglecting the neck and chest takes vengeance by wrinkling, sagging and displaying dark spots we hide with high-neck clothes. These places' skin is thinner and doesn't have a lot of blood flow, which makes it difficult for it to heal. They are areas that we often forget to protect from the sun. Use the same products that you apply on your face.

10. Remove your Makeup before Bed:
Leaving makeup and dirt on the skin clog pores and it can cause excessive dryness and even skin dandruff. A sugar-like compound that is capable of producing bacteria overnight is present in most cosmetics. Remove eye makeup completely as well, as it may result in Milia cysts, which are tiny white bumps, or scaly rashes that appear around the eyes.

11. In case you have not slept enough:
Use some soya milk to fake a good night's sleep. Natural anti-inflammatory agents relieve swelling, and soy proteins hydrate skin to minimize the appearance of dryness. Cold soya milk helps shrink

swelling and constricts veins so Mae's eyes look less reddish. To make a soothing, redness-eliminating compress, pour a small amount of soya milk into a bowl, soak two cotton balls and squeeze out the excess milk. After that, place the cotton balls for five minutes over your eyes (or any other area of your face that has red or irritated skin).

12. Clear your Swollen eyes in the Morning:

Fluid fills up under our eyes each night because we are lying down. To elevate the face when sleeping, try using two pillows. Massage away the extra fluid in the morning.

13. Avoid Hot Water:

A steamy shower may feel good, but it's one of the worst things you can do for your skin. The heat strips off essential oils and creates a mild burn. Redness results from the dilation of blood vessels as a result of an attempt to cool the skin. "Whenever you're in your twenty-somethings, a hot shower might make you feel better, but once you're in your thirties, it can take two hours. Your skin just cannot shrink back to its previous size by the time you are in your forties.

14. Moisturize Regularly:

Since skin cools naturally by evaporating water, most lotions and creams contain active chemicals that form a barrier to protect the skin's surface and keep moisture in, you still have a short while before the hydration is lost forever. Regularly apply moisturizers.

15. Be Extra Gentle when Defuzzing your Face:

Scarring or spots can result during waxing and tweezing, especially in women with darker complexions. Before shaving, clean the region with an antibacterial wash to prepare your skin. Additionally, if you want to prevent discoloration, be sure to have a post-treatment regimen that contains anti-inflammatory substances to assist the skin repair and become calmer rapidly.

16. Eat Watermelon as Snack:

Adding a lycopene-rich food, such as watermelon, helps reduce damage caused by sun exposure, prevents future wrinkling and possibly even lowers skin cancer risk. Aim for one cup each day by adding it to smoothies, salsas, and salads.

17. Exfoliate without Scrubbing: Over time, the natural enzymes in your skin work less effectively at removing dead skin cells, so they hang on and prevent your skin from shining making you look ashy and gray. Try some natural exfoliants.

18. Put on your Sunglasses: They provide more protection against under-eye wrinkling and aging than makeup. While your eyes are equipped to handle sunlight, the area around them is comprised of the thinnest skin, where you see signs of

aging. Stop the wrinkles, choose a pair of polarized glasses that's wide enough to fully cover the eye area.
19. Drink 3 Liters of Water Daily: Toxins that lead to irritation and blemishes are removed by water. Additionally, it helps to transfer nutrients and oxygen to skin cells and guards against dehydration, which can hasten the aging process. Drink 3 liters of water daily, more if you are active or live in a hot climate. Add a little flavor with a skin-soothing tea like chamomile or mint.
20. Take Caution with your Products: We are all in a hurry to see results but patience can ensure that the results you get are positive. When you're starting a new product, use it every

other day, and never try multiple new buys at once. Even with a new skincare system, introduce one product every three to four days at the least. You'll rarely experience dryness, irritation and burning. And if you do, you'll know right away the cause. Give any new product at least 12 weeks and up to 6 months to see if it's really improving your skin before stopping it.

21. Cut down on Carbs:

According to research, eating a lot of fats and carbohydrates makes you seem older. Due to the damage they inflict on our skin, creamy cheeses and fatty meats are often referred to as aging fats. To keep your cells rejuvenated, stick to lean protein like fish, white meat(poultry), beans and lentils.

22. Don't forget your Vegetables:
Look for an anti-aging cream that has plant-derived antioxidants such as mushroom or soya. When we eat plants, their anti-cancer characteristics help them survive through their digestion. "Think of what that means for their long-lasting powerful benefits when applied directly to the skin.

23. Eat your Broccoli:
They are superior to oranges. Research shows that vitamin C-rich foods mop up the free radicals that cause wrinkles and sagging and help remove the DNA damage they form. Increase your vitamin C intake for

skin protection and wound healing, and consider applying some to your skin alongside it. In one study, women who treated sun-damaged skin with a vitamin C cream for six months saw significant improvement in fine lines and discoloration.

24. Keep your hands off your Face: Picking on your skin, even lightly, can permanently damage skin. Your skin can clear up with no medications if you stop touching it. Every time you squeeze a pimple, the skin becomes inflamed and distressed. The oil cells burst at the same time as the bacterium is forced deep inside the hole, adding to the agony. The result? More acne, plus discoloration and scarring.

25. Give your Skin a Berry Tasty Treat:

Raspberries are abundant in ellagic acid, an antioxidant that helps delay the appearance of wrinkles on the skin, according to study. It prevents the sun from destroying the collagen that makes skin supple and attractive. Add in honey, it naturally holds water against the skin for maximum moisture. Try this recipe for a fine skin. Use a teaspoon of honey and a handful of raspberries to mash the mixture, and afterward use the face mask and scrub the skin for 15 to 20 minutes. Rinse and pat dry.

26. Diet:

To achieve a fair, smooth, and bright complexion from the inside out, you must consume a lot of water. Drink fruit juice to clear your blood. Eat apples, guava, pears, green vegetables, fish, eggs, nuts, oatmeal, melons, carrots etc. Amla juice and milk with a small amount of saffron should be consumed every day.

CHAPTER 12

15 NATURAL WAYS TO MAKE YOUR SKIN SOFT

1. Virgin Coconut Oil: Massage your skin with virgin coconut oil. It moisturizes and protects your skin from major types of breakouts. 3 to 4 times a week, give your skin a massage with coconut oil. Massaging your skin with virgin coconut oil mixed with vitamin E can control the aging of your skin.

2. Paste of Ripe Pawpaw: Apply it on your face or on your body, leave it for 10 to 15 minutes, then wash this with water. It will make your skin fresh and soft.

3. Banana and Liquid Milk: Mash 2 bananas, add milk to form a paste, apply this paste on your face and leave it on for 20 minutes and then rinse it off.

4. Eat Fatty Fishes like Sardine and mackerel at least one or two times per week, to provide omega-3 fatty acid which keeps your skin soft and looking young.

5. Paste of Apricot and Honey: Apply it on your skin. After waiting about ten to fifteen minutes, wash it with water. It helps to remove excess oil from your skin, reduces wrinkles and makes your skin fresh, soft and smooth.

6. Exfoliate Your Skin: Exfoliate Once a week or at least once in two

weeks. Exfoliation removes dead cells from your body and makes your skin soft and smooth.

7. Grated Carrot mixed with one spoon of Honey: Apply this all over the face and leave it for only 15 minutes. Wash off using water after ten to fifteen minutes.

8. Beans and Leafy Vegetables are important sources of Vitamin E: Vitamin E helps slow down the aging of the skin and makes your skin look younger.

9. Mixture of a Spoon of Honey, Egg, White and Grated Potato: Apply this on the face and let it dry. Wash it off with cold water to give you a smooth soft skin.

10. Honey and Rosewater: For soft and smooth skin, face and neck. Mix 1 teaspoon honey and 1 tsp rosewater. Apply as a mask. Use fresh water to rinse off after 15 minutes.

11. Strawberry mixed with sour cream: Apply the mixture on your face and neck after 30 minutes of washing with rain water or freshwater. This gives a soft skin.

12. Prepare a Facial mask with Avocado and Yogurt: Avocado contains vitamin E, as well as other natural oils and is a good moisturizer for dry skin. Yogurt is best for exfoliation and smoothness of your skin. Take a ripe avocado, peel and remove the seed, and put in a blender with four tablespoons of plain yogurt.

Blend well then gently apply on your face and neck. Remove it with lukewarm water after 15 minutes has passed.

13. A Facial Mask with Banana, Honey and Yogurt is also very effective for nourishing and moisturizing dry skin. Two bananas, one spoonful of honey, and 1/2 a cup of yogurt are required for this recipe. Put all ingredients in a blender and mix until it dries. Remove it with warm water. Yogurt hydrates and softens your dry skin, it will also exfoliate your skin, removing dead skin cells.

14. Drink Plenty of Water: Drinking 2 to 3 liters of water every day helps flush out toxins and other harmful

chemicals from your body. It also helps you to have smooth and fresh skin.

15. Ensure Regular Exercise: It helps you to tone your muscles and also prevents your skin from sagging. Exercise also improves blood circulation and skin condition. It makes your skin soft and flawless.

CHAPTER 13

HOMEMADE FAIR SKIN BEAUTY TIPS

1. Lemon is a great bleaching agent that can help you overcome your troubles with fairness and will make your face sparkle.

2. You can progressively whiten your face by employing this tip: apply potato juice to your skin.

3. You can use this easy and quick fix before attending a party. Peel a banana, take the pulp, correctly combine it, and apply it on your face to observe the amazing results. Keep the paste on your face for preferably ten to fifteen minutes.

4. You can apply papaya juice on your face to make it fair and glowing and it also removes dead cells from your skin and repairs your skin in no time.

5. Combine lemon juice and cucumber juice on your skin; this will brighten your skin and is excellent for oily skin types.

6. Take an egg, separate the white, and rub it to the surface of your face. This will help you have soft, smooth skin.

Once combined with milk, apply the paste to your skin to make it sparkle and remove dirt from the pores.

7. Grind the orange peel after drying it. Once combined with milk, apply the paste to your skin to make it

sparkle and remove dirt from the pores.

8. Curd contains zinc and lactic acid, both of which are excellent for the skin. Apply yogurt on your skin's surface to quickly achieve fairer-looking skin.

9. Use almond and olive oil to lighten your skin, clean up the pores on your face, and treat skin that is dry using this natural therapy.

10. One of the greatest methods for softening and beautifying your skin is to use rose water.

CHAPTER 14

WHAT TO DO TO LOOK NATURALLY BEAUTIFUL

1. Eat Healthy: Eat healthy foods like fish, fresh fruits and vegetables. You must eat other foods but lower the intake of fat, sugar and calories. Avoid consuming excessive amounts of junk food, such as pizza, cookies, cakes, and biscuits. Trying to lose weight by starving yourself won't work in the long run, and you run the danger of getting serious health problems. Consume a balanced diet that includes fruit, vegetables, protein, and adequate amounts of water.

2. Consume Healthy Liquids: Drink plenty of cool not cold water daily. Water removes toxins from your body and provides your skin with a healthy glow. Avoid consuming too much caffeine and limit your alcohol consumption.

3. Get Lots of Vitamin D(fresh air) and Regular Exercise: Both will make you look and feel younger. Exercise maintains fitness, releases pent-up energy that would otherwise be demanding to manage, and gives you renewed vitality. The best technique to get rid of the frown lines is through exercise. Exercise regularly to maintain your level of

fitness. Knowing whenever you're feeling your best (with neither too much nor too little activity) is important.

4. Get at least 6-8 hours of sleep each night.
You Need to Understand your Body Better to Develop your Beauty Regime.
Discover what suits you best by becoming aware of your body.
What type of skin do you have, combination, oily or dry skin?
What texture is your hair?
How does your skin react when using particular cosmetics?
By being aware of these elements, you can create a beauty routine that

maintains your attractive appearance on a natural basis. The stages that follow will assist you in learning these concepts and successfully putting them into practice.

A. Exfoliate your skin to wake it up and give you a healthy glow. Do this once a week. You may develop breakouts more frequently if you over-exfoliate.
B. Never wash your face with hot water. It makes it dry. Always use normal or cold water that energizes your skin.
C. Moisturize your skin daily. As you age, this will help to maintain your skin supple and youthful-looking. Apply moisturizer at bedtime to

prevent sweat and debris that accumulate on your skin during the day from getting trapped.

D. Steam your face regularly. Boil 1.5 liters of water until it is very hot. When you can, pour the boiling, hot water into the container as quickly as you can. Put a cloth over your head for maximum advantage and raise your face above the bowl of hot water. Your face will feel as though it is getting steamy from the intense heat. This is an effective way to get rid of blemishes and whatever scars you may have because the heat virtually kills the bacteria by forcing it to return to your skin.

E. Be sparing with makeup. Heavy makeup hides true beauty! Work on your skin instead, applying coconut oil to your face before you sleep will smooth and clear your skin tone plus it treats acne. A healthy glow can be destroyed by excessive makeup. Additionally, it teaches people to anticipate an unnatural you.

F. Try going without makeup. Allowing your skin to breathe will be better in the long run. Before going to bed, constantly wash your face with warm water and take off your makeup.

G. Take good care of your hair. Never use hot water to wash your hair; instead, use warm or lukewarm water. All the natural oils are removed with hot water. Style it according to the season so that you are at ease and your hair is shielded from the elements. Always keep your hair brushed. to maintain it there throughout the day. Use a quality shampoo and conditioner (use only organic products, if you can). To avoid over-drying the hair, avoid anything that sulfates in it.

To get rid of residue, occasionally add a little baking soda to your shampoo.

H. To have a brilliant smile, brush your teeth, whiten them, and practice proper dental hygiene. For cleaner teeth and fresher breath, think about using mouthwash and dental floss. Brush your teeth with a pinch of baking powder, salt and vinegar to make them brighter..

CHAPTER 15

MAINTAINING A NATURALLY BEAUTIFUL ATTITUDE.

1. Smile. You'll reveal a new you. Avoid drinking Pepsi, Coke, etc. Your teeth become stained, giving your grin a yellow appearance.

2. Practice daily or regular gratitude. Counting your blessings can help to keep you positive and smiling.

3. Stand tall with great posture. To feel where your shoulders should be, roll them around a few times. Keep your head high. Avoid adopting a "forward-head posture" by keeping your head level on your shoulders.

4. Be confident. If you're not. Try some assertiveness training and affirmations. Remind yourself frequently that you are and consistently will be attractive.

5. Seek to be happy with who you are. This can take time to learn and it can be buffeted now and then by events in life but try to make this your grounded point and always return to enjoying your current self as well as your past self and your future self.

6. Never say you're not pretty, that will make you upset. Always be self-assured and think positively; your poise and tone will reflect this.

7. Use clothes you feel good in, and that define your features. Avoid donning attire that does not enhance

your physique. You don't need to religiously stick to every single fashion tip you come across but do take the time to learn how to bring out the beauty of your unique figure. Wear some matching accessories with your dress to give you a pretty and modern look.

8. Don't worry and rush around too much. Take at least ten minutes a day to do something you find relaxing.

9. Avoid makeup that contains a lot of chemicals. Choose natural products instead, and employ them sparingly.

10. Putting Vaseline on your eyelashes (and eyebrows, if necessary) every night for a month or more will condition them, inducing them to grow more and shine.

11. If you want to have long eyelashes without using fake ones, try adding mascara.

Warnings:

1. Do not use harsh cleansers or astringents on your skin, use natural oils and honey to gently moisturize and cleanse the face.

2. Check to make sure that you are not allergic to any kind of makeup before using it. Don't compare yourself to others.

3. Do not pull and tug at your skin. Avoid touching your skin when you are going about your daily activities. When you are cleaning your skin, use gentle massaging movements.

CHAPTER 16

10 NATURAL BEAUTY TRICKS USING COOKING INGREDIENTS

1. Sugar Skin Care.

Artificial products are easy to try but they sometimes contain harsh chemicals. Natural substances in your kitchen are sometimes very good for you. A multi-purpose item like sugar can serve you in ways you never thought about. Mix a few tablespoons of sugar with water and a paste. Apply this to wet skin and leave it on for a few minutes, then rinse with cool water. Use cocoa butter as a moisturizer.

2. Green Tea Spray.
Recipe: 1 green tea bag, spray bottle
Method: Use a green tea bag and boiling water to make tea as you normally would then set it aside to cool. Once it has cooled, put it in a spray bottle and place it in the refrigerator. When you come back from being out in the sun for a long time, spray it on your skin as a refresher and to help reverse sun damage. Bonus- Put the used tea bag in the freezer and once it's cold, use it on your eyes to help reduce puffiness.

3. Raw Brown Sugar and Honey Scrub

Recipe: 1 tablespoon of honey, half cup of raw brown sugar, Grapeseed oil.

Method: Mix the honey and brown sugar, and add about 3 drops of Grapeseed oil. Clean skin should be scrubbed with this mixture, applied, and then removed with warm water. The honey acts as an exfoliator, while the Grapeseed oil conditions and softens the skin.

4. Apple Cider Vinegar Bath

Recipe: Half a cup of apple cider vinegar. 1/3 cup of sunflower oil.

Method: Get lukewarm or warm water in a bath, add apple cider vinegar and sunflower oil. Soak yourself in it. Apple cider vinegar baths are ideal for those who suffer from issues of extremely dry skin with itchy patches, like those caused by conditions like eczema and psoriasis. The vinegar offers relief to the uncomfortable patches while the sunflower oil soothes and softens the skin. Since the water is warm instead of hot it avoids further irritation or scalding already inflamed skin tissue.

5. Bentonite Clay Detox Mask

You can obtain bentonite clay from health stores.

Recipe: Bentonite Clay, 2 tablespoons of apple cider vinegar, any essential oil.

Method: Create a soft mixture using the Bentonite clay, and apple cider vinegar (if you have sensitive skin, substitute 2 tablespoons of sour cream for the vinegar) and rub on the skin. Let it dry completely. While it is drying, it is normal to feel a pulsating sensation, No worries, it is the mask blast pulling those irritating toxins that your skin appear red, Apply Grapeseed or sweet almond oil and let your skin rest.

6. Oil Cleansing; for Soft Skin
Instead of using harsh soap, clean your skin with castor oil mixed with olive, coconut, or almond oil. This will cleanse your skin naturally and will not pull out natural oils. A good

blend is 25% Castor oil(never use alone) and 75% sweet almond oil.
Method: Apply a little oil to a dry face and rub it into the skin for some time. To take off, place a clean washcloth over your face and hold it there until it begins to cool. Wipe your face with the washcloth gently until all of the oil is removed.

7. Food Facial Mask
Many foods you eat as breakfast are also beneficial for your skin.
How: Create a fantastic toning mask for the face that keeps skin shining by combining honey, plain yogurt, or whipped egg whites.

8. Naturally White Teeth.

Use strawberries and baking soda as an effective, natural teeth whitener. Teeth can be whitened via oil pulling, which involves swishing oil about in one's mouth and then throwing it out. How to Do It: Make a paste of equal parts mashed strawberries and baking soda. For up to 30 minutes, place a mouthguard or dental tray on the teeth. Repeat a couple of times per week until you have the whitest possible results for your teeth. To speed things up swish with 1 Tablespoon of olive oil each night for 20 minutes and then spit and brush well. This helps remove toxins and you can vouch for its whitening effect also.

9. Natural Hair Conditioner

For an occasional hair-strengthening treat, mix some other breakfast foods into a natural hair mask. Use little, but it keeps hair smooth and shiny and even helps on extremely curly hair.

How to Do it: Mix one banana and one avocado and purée until smooth (a good way to use over-ripe bananas and avocados). Add essential oils for Fragrance. Put on a shower cap after brushing your clean, damp hair. At least fifteen minutes should be left on.

10. Sugar Scrub

Sugar is not good for your body. It is great for your skin! Sugar is a fantastic technique to tighten up and smooth skin since unlike your fat cells, your skin doesn't metabolize or store glucose or fructose.

How to Do It: Combine equal amounts of white or brown sugar with almond or olive oil, then flavor with your preferred essential oils. Massage the mixture into the skin for a few minutes to exfoliate it. Rinse off with warm water.

CHAPTER 17

SPECIAL NATURAL BEAUTY METHODS FOR BLACK SKIN

Cocoa Butter:

Cocoa butter is a natural moisturizer. It reduces the appearance of stretch marks and smooths rough elbows and knees. Use cocoa butter twice a day for best results. Pure cocoa butter can be found at health food stores.

Natural Exfoliant:

To reveal a new layer of smooth, young skin, exfoliate your skin. Put a few tablespoons of coarse sea salt in a bowl and add enough orange juice to make a paste. In gentle circular motions, apply to the skin. Rinse with cool water to tighten pores. Moisturize with cocoa butter to complete the facial.

Homemade Honey Smoother:
For smooth, beautiful skin use a honey moisturizer. Mix equal amounts of honey and plain yogurt in a bowl. Apply generously to the skin while bathing or in the shower. Rinse well after 5 to 10 minutes. Apply a moisturizer after this treatment.

CHAPTER 18

HOW TO USE CURRY LEAF FOR BEAUTY TREATMENTS

Curry leaves are slightly bitter and very aromatic. Their mineral and vitamin content are calcium, phosphorus, iron, niacin, Vitamin B3 and vitamin C.

1. To prevent Premature Graying: Eat a large quantity of curry leaves. The leaves have the property to nourish the hair roots so that new hair roots that grow are healthier with normal pigment.

2. Hair Tonic: Boil a handful of Curry leaves and Marudhani or Mehendi leaves in coconut oil till they are

reduced to a blackened residue. The oil forms an excellent hair tonic to stimulate hair growth and retain the natural pigmentations.

3. To Treat Burns and Bruises: Curry leaves can be effectively used to treat burns, bruises, and skin eruptions. Apply as a plaster over the areas affected.

4. To Prevent Eye Disorders: Fresh juice of curry leaves suffused in the eyes makes them look bright. It also prevents the early development of cataracts.

HOW TO USE CORIANDER (CILANTRO) FOR REMEDIES

Cilantro is the leaf of coriander herb used as a tea for both urinary tract infections and for headaches. The power of cilantro to keep food fresh is increased when it is combined with onion or garlic. It is also believed to give sexual stamina.

Cilantro is tasty and it is antimicrobial. The essential oils in cilantro are effective against bacteria and also slow the growth of E. coli and Salmonella. Cilantro contains flavonoids and phenols which aids digestion and relieves upset stomach. Coriander and manna are both analogies made in the Bible. Cilantro is used to garnish various dishes. Traditional medicine has utilized coriander seeds to treat sleeplessness and anxiety since they are believed to have antimicrobial characteristics. Coriander is made into a powder after roasting. Taking coriander as tea helps to clear the body of lead, mercury and aluminum.

1. Scientific investigations have verified its therapeutic properties, including the management of cholesterol, and blood sugar, and the generation of free radicals. To treat rheumatism and soothe sore joints, use a coriander seed poultice.

2. Throat pain can be relieved by chewing on a few coriander and black pepper seeds frequently.

3. Eye infection: For relief from the agony of conjunctivitis, the cooled decoration of coriander powder can be used as an eye wash.

4. Digestion: Soak one teaspoon of coriander or dhania seeds and one teaspoon of desiccated and powdered amla seeds overnight, add honey and eat early morning on an empty stomach for headache and stomach ache. This will also increase appetite.

5. Body odor: To limit body odor, add one teaspoon of coriander powder and two teaspoons of Amla or Gooseberry powder to a glass of water and drink two to three times a day.

6. Menstrual problems: Crush cilantro leaves and extract juice. Add a little camphor and 10 to 15 cc of juice. To stop excessive menstrual bleeding, take up to three times daily.

7. Joint pain: Mix powders of method seeds and ajwain with coriander seed powder in equal quantities. Drink to ease the pain in osteoarthritis.

8. Cough: 5 tablespoons of ground coriander seed mixed with half a bottle of honey is an excellent cough suppressant.

9. High-blood pressure: Soak one tablespoon of coarsely ground coriander seeds in a cup of filtered

water overnight. Filter out the seed the next morning. To this add a spoonful of sugar candy powder and drink it early in the morning.

10. Morning sickness: To a glass of rice-washed water, add a spoonful of coriander seed powder mixed with equal sugar-sweet powder. Drink it early in the morning.

11. Urinary infection: Soak coarse coriander powder in boiled but cooled water overnight. Filter before drinking in the morning.

12. Induces perspiration and helps with digestion: This is what Chinese medicine says about coriander in

addition to being warm, pungent and positively affecting the lungs and spleen.

13. Halitosis and bad breath; Coriander is also used to cure these conditions in general. A tea made with coriander will eliminate colds, and stomach aches and help with excessive gastric acid problems. Coriander is not for You: If you have cracked lips or heavy thirst. Regular consumption of coriander will reduce the smell of urine due to internal heat.

CHAPTER 19

HOW TO REMOVE DARK SPOTS AND PATCHES FROM THE SKIN

1. HOW YOU CAN REMOVE DARK SKIN ON THE BACK:

A darkish patch on the back could be a big problem for ladies especially those who wear blouses. The cause may be exposure to the sun. Sometimes ladies who are not outgoing have it. The dark shade also is seen around the neck. You can try this natural solution. This treatment requires consistency to cure it completely. The first step is to apply coconut oil or your favorite oil. But coconut oil has a rejuvenating effect. Massage well on the back till the oil gets applied thoroughly. Then grind almond seeds to powder. Mix it with half the quantity of sandalwood powder. Then add milk and make a paste. Juice from a couple of lemons should be added. Apply this almond pack on the back. Application of this pack should be given in round movements. Leave the pack for about 10 to 15 minutes. Then wash it off. Expect gradual but visible results even from the first trial. Repeat daily for full results.

2. DARK LIPS

Dark lips may be a minute but disturbing problem. This may be due to various reasons. The face may be fair but if the lips are dark the total fairness may be affected. Try this simple remedy. Mix equal quantities of coconut oil and almond oil and apply it on your lips. You can also mix honey and vaseline and apply it on your lips. Applying this for a few weeks cures it. This is something you can do whenever it suits you. But remember to leave for about 10 minutes minimum.

3. DARK SHADE ON THE SIDE OF THE NOSE

This may be due to the use of spectacles. Apply a mixture of coconut oil and almond oil on the affected area to remove the black mark. After 30 min, wipe it off with a wet cotton ball. Do it for a few weeks.

4. TO GET RID OF DARK CIRCLES UNDER THE EYES

Combine 1 tsp of groundnut oil and some lime juice and apply it regularly under the eye to eradicate dark circles under the eyes.

CHAPTER 20

FIGHTING ACNE AND PIMPLES; NATURAL CURES

1. Pimple treatment

Use this quick fix only as needed. If you do get an open wound, you should allow it to cure naturally. However, there are times when you need the pimple gone now. This solution will help make it go away in a day or two.

You Need: Baking soda Honey (preferred), Lemon juice.

Apply a small amount of baking soda, wet using water, honey (recommended), lemon juice on the pimple in the evening after washing your face. The amount should be sufficient to cover the pimple. Pop a little Band-Aid on top. In the morning, it should be a lot less noticeable or even gone. If it becomes more swollen, wash your face and then apply an ice cube to lessen the swelling. Only a couple of nights' worth of therapy is required to get rid of the zit. Keep that area clean with witch hazel.

Teenagers who have pimples have the worst condition in terms of skin care. When there are many pimples, the face appears ugly. Along with having a horrible appearance, pimples also have a bad texture. Sometimes, it causes facial skin perforations. This causes mental worry to teens. Several products on the market promise instantaneous healing. But most of the time the experience from the store-bought products are not that much favorable. Additionally, it occasionally causes adverse effects. It causes skin damage etc. It is perfectly normal to choose a reliable home remedy at this time to treat acne. Since it's natural, there won't be any negative effects. Here is an all-natural home cure that uses tulsi and neem leaves.

Neem leaf (Azadirachta indica (leaves and fruit)
It is highly medicinal. This is used for several skin problems. Here we need

a few fresh leaves. Take 5 to 10 leaves depending on the purpose.
Tulsi leaf (Ocimum tenuiflorum)
Tulsi is also used for several skin disorders. Here we need 5 leaves.
Preparation of Pimples cures home remedy:
You need Neem and tulsi leaves in the proportion 1:2. Use five neem leaves in addition to your 10 tulsi leaves. For this use 6 tulsi leaves and 3 neem leaves. Mash the leaves to make a paste, and add a few drops of water.

Application; Wash the face well with water. Wipe the excess water from the face. Use the paste ONLY where the pimple is. Apply thickly on the pimples. There may be some burning feelings but don't worry. Wash it off after 10-15 minutes of waiting. The neem leaf is the primary component in this dish. As a result, you can increase the amount of neem leaves used the next day if there is no discomfort. However, if you have discomfort, you must consume fewer neem leaves the following day. Do this every day for five days in a row, and then once every three to four days until the pimples are gone. This pimple-cure home remedy is safe and effective.

Keep Acne or Pimples in Check.

Stop acne before it spoils your beauty. Try these pimple-prevention tips.

1. Change your pillowcase every four or five days. A new, bacteria-free pillowcase can stop your skin from erupting overnight.
2. Keep your hands off your face. Stop fidgeting with your face or frequently resting your lower jaw in your palm. Even modest amounts of the oils on the skin of your hands can result in outbreaks.
3. Tie your hair back while you sleep. Keep your long hair away from your face while you're sleeping. Be sure to keep hair off your forehead.
4. Get your beauty rest. Make sure you're rested and relaxed because stress might cause breakouts.
5. If you use birth control (females). Be aware that some contraceptives

containing estrogen have effect breakouts. Find out if this is the right choice for you.

6. Do not pick or pop pimples. It can make it worse and lead to permanent scarring.

CHAPTER 21

REMOVING DARK CIRCLES UNDER THE EYES

First, Clean your Eyes. The best cleansing agent is water. Fresh Milk is also a good eye cleanser. A Clean Cotton ball can be dipped in milk and can be applied to the eyes. At work during meal intervals splash your eyes with pure water because water not only makes your eyes have Clear Vision but also gives your Eyes a Fresh Look. Grate a carrot and combine it thoroughly with a spoonful of honey. Apply this all over the face and leave it for only 15 minutes. Wash off with water after ten to fifteen minutes. You may use this every week regularly. This can be used by all skin types and make your skin soft and smooth.

PORES ON THE FACE

Try this very simple remedy to diminish the appearance of open pores. Mix three tsp. tomato pulp and one tsp. of multani mitti(clay) and apply it on the affected areas for a few weeks. This will reduce the appearance of open pores.

HAIR TREATMENT FOR NATURAL SHEEN

Is your hair wavy or kinky? Does your hair lose shine? Did you lose the natural sheen of your hair? Whatever may be the reason, now you need a hair treatment to recover the shine and sheen of your hair. A shine-boosting mask that moisturizes your hair can be helpful to you.

HAIR TREATMENT WITH AVOCADO HAIR MASK

Take 1/2 avocado, 1/2 ripe banana, 1 tbsp yogurt, and 1 tablespoon olive oil. Put all the ingredients in a mixer and make it a paste. Apply it to your hair. Put on a shower cap and wait for 20 minutes. Wash it off with water. If you feel like using shampoo, then any mild shampoo. Condition the next day. This hair treatment gives extra moisturizing and Avocado is a good deep conditioner also.

This hair treatment can be done once a week.

TO TREAT DRY HAIR

2 tsp long pepper (Piper longum), 2 tsp Fenugreek seeds and some poppy seeds soak them in a cow's milk and grind them together and apply it on the hair. Keep for 20 minutes and rinse off to make your hair soft.

AVOCADO-CARROT CREAM FACE MASK

You are all aware of the benefits of carrots and avocados. But it's also highly beneficial to your skin. Your skin is nourished and made smooth and lustrous by the avocado's pulp. Beta carotene is included in carrots, which can improve the complexion of your skin.

Ingredients: Smashed avocado- 1 Boiled and smashed carrot, 5 tsp Cooked-oats.

THE RIGHT WAY TO MAKE AN AVOCADO CARROT CREAM FACE MASK.

Put all of the ingredients in a mixer jar and blend them to a paste. Add a little water if needed. The mask is ready to use.

How to Apply: Wash your face with normal water. Then cover your entire face and neck with the mask. Avoid the eye area. Wait for 20 minutes and wash it off with cool water. You can repeat this once a week after performing it daily for the first several days. Your skin's appearance will change noticeably as a result.

PAWPAW FACE MASK

Refreshing Face Mask with Pawpaw, Milk and Sandalwood Powder. Pawpaw gives a light bleaching effect and glow. Milk adds special smoothness to facial skin. Sandalwood makes your skin extra beautiful. All are natural.

Ingredients: 5 tsp mashed pawpaw, 1 tsp. sandalwood powder, 3tsp. milk powder.

How to Apply Face Mask:

Add sandalwood powder and milk powder to the pawpaw paste and mix well with a spoon. Then wash the face with normal water and apply a mask all over the face, wait for 10-15 minutes. Then wash it off using cold water. All types of skin can use it. But for extremely dry skin, apply your favorite oil before applying the mask. Once in a week is sufficient to give good results. If you react to any of the ingredients, avoid using it.

CHAPTER 22

HOW TO USE FRUITS AND VEGETABLES TO CURE SKIN PROBLEMS

1. Lemon Juice Scrub

Mix lemon juice mixed with pure honey and granulated sugar. Apply it in a circular pattern to your face using clean fingers or cotton wool. This natural scrub will remove dead cells from your face giving a radiant glow. Additionally, you can use this mixture on your lips and as an overall body cleanse.

2. Cucumber

Applying a paste made from mashed cucumber and raw milk will improve your complexion. Get rid of the green skin, chop the cucumber into smaller pieces, and mash with a fork. Leave it on your skin for about 15 minutes, then wash off with fresh water. It also helps in soothing and softening your skin.

3. Tomatoes

Tomatoes are good antioxidants. For wrinkles-free skin, mash two large tomatoes and apply them evenly on your face. After 20 minutes, thoroughly rinse with cold water. Tomatoes are also great for oily skin. They are great for the skin as they have cooling and astringent properties. They are naturally acidic thereby helping to balance the skin and get rid of excessive oil. Evenly apply tomato pulp on your face. Let it dry for 15 minutes and wash your face with warm water.

4. Cucumber and Lemon to Remove Blemishes

Now you can stay away from painful blackhead extraction during facials that often injure the skin and leave dark scars. Prepare a paste using equal parts the juice of a cucumber and lemon juice to make a paste for fairer skin tone and natural blackhead removal (use a blender, small mortar, or simply a fork). Apply this paste to your face and neck before taking a bath. Let your skin absorb it for at least ten minutes. With regular use, you will notice fewer blackheads and a fairer skin tone.

5. Do Justice to Water and Sleep
Sound sleep and water are natural facial beauty enhancers. 3 liters of water per day and 6 to 8 hours of sleep daily are essential for the skin to revitalize and repair damaged tissues. Do things you enjoy to burst stress and reduce the likelihood of having stress-induced acne breakouts.

CHAPTER 23

8 NATURAL WAYS TO GIVE YOU ATTRACTIVE EYES

Eyes are the most conspicuous feature of one's Personality. It doesn't matter if you have large or small eyes; nonetheless, exhausted and swollen eyes may lessen your personality, while shining, attractive eyes may increase it by giving you a captivating appearance. To have attractive and charming eyes you don't need to spend a lot of money on chemical products because you can make your eyes attractive and impressive just by following some tips which are given below.

1. First, Clean your Eyes. The best cleansing agent is water. Fresh Milk is also a good Eye Cleanser. Dip a Clean Cotton ball in milk and apply it on your Eyes.

2. One or Two Drops of Pure Rose Water can increase the Glow of Your Eyes.

3. Proper Sleep: At least 6 to 8 hours is also essential for your Eyes.

4. You can massage your EyeBrows and eyelashes with glycerin to maintain the Density of your EyeBrows and EyeLashes, giving your Eyes an Attractive Look.

5. Protect your Eyes from Harmful Sun Rays by Using Sunglasses.

6. Eat a Diet Rich in vitamins A, C and E. Eat Green Vegetables, Citrus

Fruits and Dairy Products Containing Calcium.

7. From time to time Splash your Eyes with Pure water because water not only makes your eyes have Clear Vision But also gives your Eyes a Fresh Look.

8. Use Cucumber Slices to Remove Dark Circles Under Eyes. Cucumber Removes Dark Circles Under Eyes. Cucumber Removes Dark Circles, helps remove Eyes Redness and diminishes Dryness of the skin under the Eyes. To apply Cucumber Slice, Lie Down on your Back then apply thin Slices of purely natural products. They Favor Wild Rose Oil.

CHAPTER 24

HOW TO NATURALLY GET RID OF BLACKHEADS ON THE FACE AND NOSE.

Blackheads are tiny, dark spots that appear on the surface of your skin. Blackheads are blocked pores (hair follicles) in the skin that are filled with skin debris or keratin and sebum, an oily substance. Blackheads occur mainly on the face and nose, a common problem among adolescents with oily skin. Blackheads can be called first-stage acne before bacteria enters the clogged pores.

CAUSES OF BLACKHEADS
Stress

- Hormonal changes
- Inheritance
- Unclean skin
- Cosmetics
- Smoking
- Alcohol
- Caffeine.

NATURAL WAYS TO CLEAR BLACKHEADS

1. Blackheads are dried out by the natural antibacterial qualities of Tomatoes. Take a small tomato, peel and smash, then apply it over the blackheads before going to bed. After leaving it overnight, rinse your face

with lukewarm water when you wake up.

2. Another all-natural item that works well to treat blackheads is lemon. Add salt to a bowl along with a few droplets of lemon juice and stir thoroughly. Apply the mixture to the blackheads after washing your face with warm water. After 20 minutes, rinse your face with warm water once more.

3. After leaving the toothpaste on the blackheads for 25 minutes, gently wash your face with warm water. For two weeks, use this solution daily to get rid of blackheads.

4. Honey has properties that work wonders for oily skin and blackheads. After 15 minutes, wash the afflicted

area with warm water and apply honey again.

5. Prepare a paste by combining baking soda and water. To get rid of the oil and filth that lead to blackheads, carefully apply the affected area, let it dry for a short while, and then wash it off with some warm water.

6. Oatmeal and yogurt are beneficial for the skin and can help clear blackheads. Mix 2 tablespoons of oatmeal with 3 tablespoons of yogurt, add 1 tablespoon of lemon juice and olive oil to it, and mix all these ingredients to form a paste. Apply the mixture to your face, let it sit for 10 to 15 minutes, then rinse with cold water.

7. Blackheads can be eliminated at home with raw eggs. One or two egg whites and one spoonful of honey should be mixed. Apply this combination to the blackhead-affected region, let it sit for 30 minutes, then rinse with warm water.

8. Prepare a mixture of equal parts of cinnamon powder and lime juice to form a thick paste. Apply the paste to the affected parts and leave on overnight, then wash off your face with warm water in the morning.

BLACKHEAD REMOVAL

There are other manual ways to remove blackheads. Here is a very simple method to remove blackheads.

Mix mint leaf paste and white camphor and apply on the affected area only. After 10-15 minutes, wipe off with a wet cotton ball by pressing gently. This may give an itching or burning sensation for those who have very sensitive skin, so take care.

CHAPTER 25

10 NATURAL WAYS TO STOP HEAVY MENSTRUAL BLEEDING

Hormonal dysregulation, irregular blood coagulation, and occasionally uterine lining abnormalities can all contribute to excessive menstrual bleeding. During the menstrual cycle, heavy bleeding is common in teenage girls with hormonal imbalances and women approaching menopause. If your menstrual cycle lasts more than a week or you have to change your sanitary pad every couple of hours, then it is a case of menorrhagia or excessive bleeding. However, you can cure this problem by following some natural tips but in case of severe condition, you may need to see a Gynecologist or doctor.

1. Banana flower is an excellent cure for heavy bleeding. Take one banana flower and cook it with a cup of fresh curd to increase the quantity of progesterone and decrease the bleeding.

2. Coriander seeds significantly lessen menstrual bleeding. Boil 20 grams of coriander seed in two cups (about 200ml) of water. Allow the water to cool after it has been reduced to a quarter of its original volume.

3. Mango bark: A mixture prepared by adding 10 ml of liquid extract of

mango bark in 139 ml of water is very effective in treating heavy bleeding. Each hour, consume a single teaspoon of this mixture. The juice of fresh mango bark is a natural home remedy to cure heavy menstrual bleeding.

4. Magnesium helps to reduce menstrual bleeding. Food rich in magnesium like sesame seeds, watermelon seeds, oats, cocoa, pumpkin, and squash must be included in the diet to cure heavy menstrual bleeding.

5. Herbal teas like chamomile tea help to cure the problem.

6. Ginger helps a lot to reduce heavy bleeding. Menstrual flow can be stopped and comfort is provided by

an infusion made by smashing and cooking ginger inside of water for a short period. To make the infusion taste better, it could be sweetened with honey or sugar. After every meal, you may absorb this infusion.

7. Mustard seeds are quite effective at reducing severe bleeding. To make a fine powder, dry mill 40 grams of mustard seeds. Use two grams of mustard seed powder in combination with milk twice a day, either before or during your period, to lessen heavy bleeding. It is an effective home remedy for heavy menstrual bleeding.

8. Combine 1/2 tsp. of ground cinnamon with a cup of boiling water. Consumption of cinnamon is one of the best home remedies to cure heavy

bleeding. You can also drink cinnamon tea to control the heavy menstrual cycle.

9. Parsley juice is also known to stop heavy bleeding.

10. Take 1-2 tablespoons of gooseberry juice with honey on an empty stomach.

OTHER THINGS YOU SHOULD DO

- Drink at least 3 liters of water daily to remove toxins from the body.

- Foods rich in iron are effective cures for the problem

- Avoid intense and heavy exercise during the condition.

- Do not eat hot and spicy food.

- Avoid refined food products such as sugar, sweets and alcohol.

CHAPTER 26

THE BEST WAY TO POSTPONE MENSTRUAL PERIODS THAT ARE ALWAYS ON TIME

Sometimes you may like to delay your menstrual periods for a few days for various reasons, maybe you have to travel. To delay the periods temporarily, try eating roasted chickpeas. Eating a handful of plain dalia dal every morning will delay periods by 3-4 days. Start this at least 5 days before your period is due. It has to be continuous. Do not break even a single day.

CHAPTER 27

SOME USEFUL NATURAL EYE CARE TIPS

Eyes Dark Circles

"Eyes Dark Circles" that give people an old and ugly look are common in both Males and Females but more noticeable in Females.

Causes:

- Extremely Tensed Conditions
- Working till late at night
- Lack of Sleep.

You begin to see Dark Circles Under the Eyes because the Skin Under the Eyes is the most sensitive and thinnest part of our skin, it has no fat deposit. Overwork, poor diet and

Sleepless hours makes the muscles of this skin tired, creating wrinkles and dark circles under the eyes.

11 WAYS TO REMOVE DARK CIRCLES UNDER THE EYES.

1. Using Cucumber Slices; Cucumber Removes Dark Circles, Eyes Redness and reduces Dryness of the Skin under the Eyes. To apply Cucumber Slices on your eyes, lie down flat on your back then place thin slices of cucumber on your eyes, be sure they touch the skin under your eyes. After 10 minutes remove them. Be careful of cucumber water and never let it enter your eyes.

2. Take half cucumber and 1 medium-sized potato then peel them off and cut them into small slices. A single tablespoon of lemon juice as well as 1/2 teaspoon of turmeric powder should be added. Now mix all ingredients in a grinder or mixer to make a thick paste. Apply this paste now to your dark circles, let it sit for 15 minutes, and then wash it off with clean water. For quick results, before going to sleep don't forget to apply almond oil on dark circles.

3. A mixture of almond oil and honey: Apply it on the affected area every night before bedtime. You will see a remarkable improvement within two or three weeks.

4. Use of tea bags reduces dark circles under the eyes because caffeine present in tea bags diminishes bulges under the eyes. Take a used tea bag but make sure it has been cooled then place it on your eyes for at least 10 minutes. But be careful and don't allow tea water to go into your eyes.

5. Make a paste of fresh mint leaves and add a few drops of lime juice to it. In a period of two to three weeks, the combination should start to show results when applied to the eyes and circles of darkness for 10-15 minutes each day.

6. Soak a cloth in hot water and apply it on affected areas for 5-10 minutes. Similarly, soak another cloth in cold

water and apply it on dark circles for the same time period. Then gently apply almond oil under the dark circles.

7. Avoid Smoking because it not only weak your Eyesight but can also constrict and damage your blood vessels and create lots of problems for blood passing through them especially blood capillaries under the eyes are so thin and delicate that if they have been constricted because of over smoking then blood has to face difficulty in passing through them.

8. Rose water is considered a natural coolant for the body and is very effective in curing dark circles. The afflicted eye area should be gently massaged for five to six minutes

using a cotton ball dipped in two or three drops of rose water. Within two to three weeks, the outcome will be visible.

9. Potato juice is also considered very effective for curing dark circles under the eyes. On the dark circles, use potato juice-soaked cotton balls for 15 minutes. Throughout that time, keep your eyes closed.

10. Eat fruits rich in antioxidants. Increase your intake of vitamin C and eat fruits like oranges, pineapple, apples, limes, guava, lemons, pawpaw, strawberries, broccoli, tomatoes, brussel sprouts, cabbage, potatoes, kale, spinach (palak), and watercress is also good sources of vitamin C.

11. Drink lots of Water as an essential part of your diet. Don't drink less than 3 liters because water is quite helpful in releasing of body's wastes and keeping eyes fresh. Besides water, also try to drink juices of tomato, carrot and mint because these juices are also considered best to reduce eyes' dark circles.

CHAPTER 28

HERBS FOR HEALING EYE WASHES

Calendula

Calendula blossoms have antibacterial and antiviral properties and can be especially effective when used on the skin and in your eyes. If your eyes are inflamed or irritated because of allergic or conjunctivitis, use an infusion of calendula and warm water as an eyewash. Because it is one of the most gentle herbs available, it will not aggravate sensitive eyes or skin.

Goldenseal

Golden is a potent herb that has antibacterial and anti-inflammatory properties. Its basic compound called berberine, is particularly effective in treating herpes simplex virus in the eyes. It's useful as an eyewash for styes and conjunctivitis. It is also an alternative to eye drops that are commercially sold to ease and soothe tired or itchy eyes. Goldenseal may irritate your eyes, so start with a weak solution for an eyewash. Make a tincture of goldenseal and water, with more water than goldenseal.

Coriander

Coriander is another herb with extensive healing properties that is ideal for an eyewash. Dried coriander is recommended for treating eye pain and irritation caused by conjunctivitis. It helps relieve pain or swelling. Create an eyewash by combining warm water and dried coriander, the fresher the better.

CHAPTER 29

NATURAL BEAUTY SECRETS FROM OTHER COUNTRIES

Women in other parts of the world have their own natural beauty materials and local secrets that they use.

FROM PORTUGAL

Natural Beauty Ingredient: Turmeric. It not only has amazing healing properties but it's an excellent beauty product. Turmeric Face Mask: Mix flour, turmeric, honey and milk to make a paste, apply it in a thin layer to your face, let it dry for 20 minutes and rinse in the shower.

The country's best beauty secrets: A beautiful seaside coast that heals the soul, wonderful weather that gives vitamin D (and a beautiful glow!) and delicious Portuguese red wines. Their healthy diet staple: The Mediterranean diet: garlic, olive oil, oranges, apples, lots of greens and fish.

FROM KOREA

Natural Beauty Ingredient: Girls have a cucumber massage when their skin gets dry. It's simple: They slice cucumbers thin and put it on a clean face. It makes the skin so.

FROM THE US

Natural Beauty Ingredient: Coconut oil. They use it for hair, skin and teeth whitening. Our country's best beauty secret: it's not exactly unique to the US but drinking water is the foundation for any beauty regime. Healthy Diet Staple: "Kale!"

CONCLUSION

Artificiality is encroaching on all areas of our life. We no longer have regard for natural things. People believe there are no simple and inexpensive natural beauty methods. We try every product that claims to make us more beautiful. Little wonder that the beauty industry in Nigeria is worth billions of Naira. According to UK survey, women will spend well over a year of their total lifespan applying make-up and beauty products that contain unregulated toxic chemicals. It appears the world is saying we cannot be beautiful unless we spend lots of time, and lots of money and risk our health, that is not true. You don't need to invest in expensive lotions to be attractive. The whole idea of beauty is about unmasking the real person, not covering it up with makeup. There are diverse ways to appreciate your body, feel more beautiful and all at little or no cost at all and it is easier to look gorgeous by just adopting some natural beauty habits and eating right. This book gives you hundreds of such beauty ideas. They are easy. They are all-natural. Make you become more beautiful.

ABOUT THE AUTHOR

Timothy M. Ross of Grace Empire Ministries is full time pastor and also teaches longevity on invitation. He was born by Long Livers and mentored by Long Livers. He has a strong obsession for longevity. These factors motivated him to become an explorer, investigator and writer on longevity related matters. He has authored many books on long life. He is a regular speaker in longevity Conferences. The author observed that though everyone, male or female desires longevity, the women folks in addition to long life also wish to look attractive. Artificial beauty products contain harsh chemicals with serious health risks. Whatever you put on your body outside ultimately enters into the body, so why put on your body what you cannot put in your mouth. To help you unmask your natural beauty, the author has researched and compiled over 360 natural beauty methods in use all over the world. Using natural products for beauty is a better option…

www.ingramcontent.com/pod-product-compliance
Lightning Source LLC
Chambersburg PA
CBHW050805260726
48660CB00004B/1263